Cesarean with a Sibling

ISBN: 9780615366470

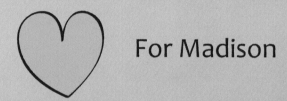 For Madison

Today is a very special day.
Mommy is coming home from
the hospital and
she's bringing
our new baby!

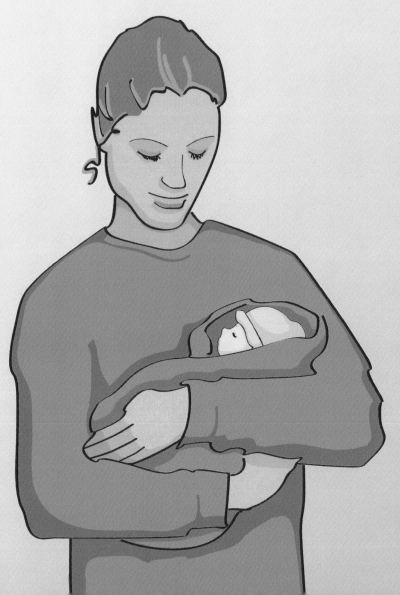

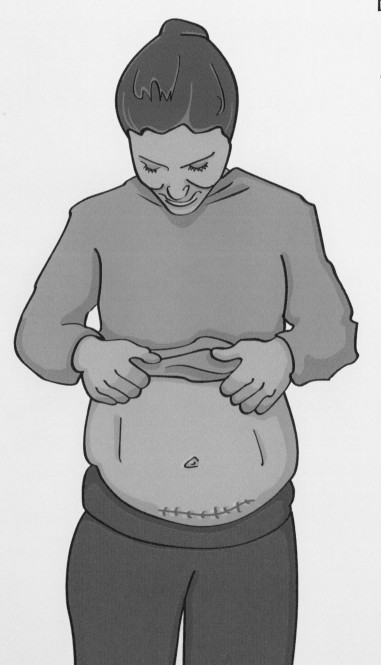

We must be gentle with
the new baby and we must
be gentle with mommy.

Mommy has a boo-boo
on her belly.

Mommy needs to rest to get better.

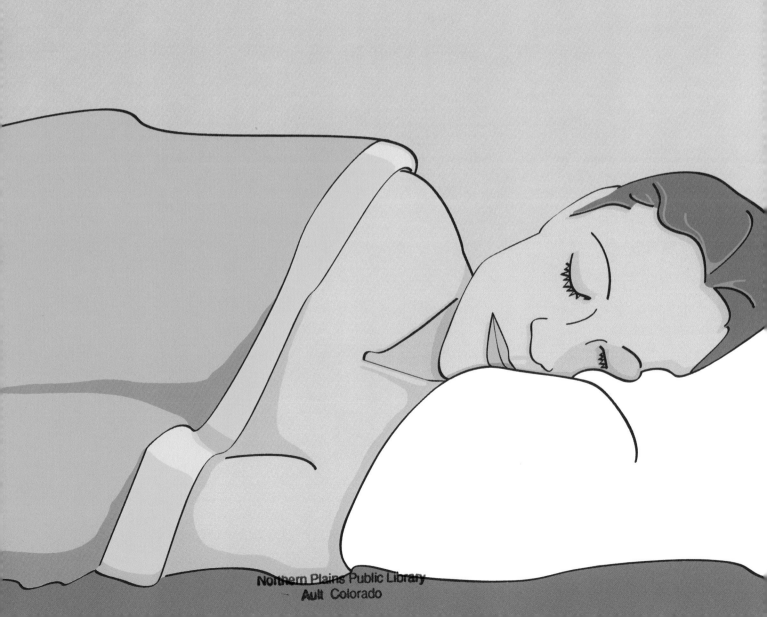

The doctor says no climbing or jumping on mommy.

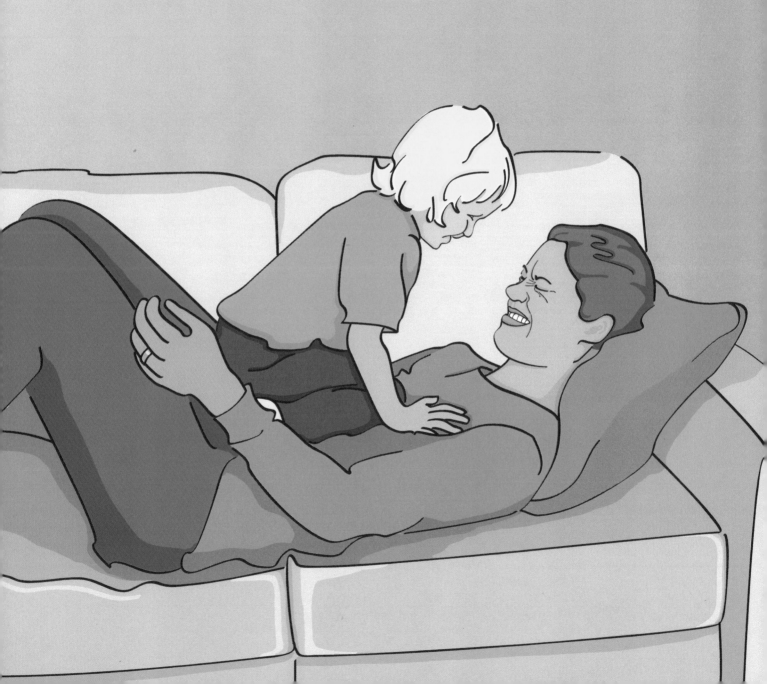

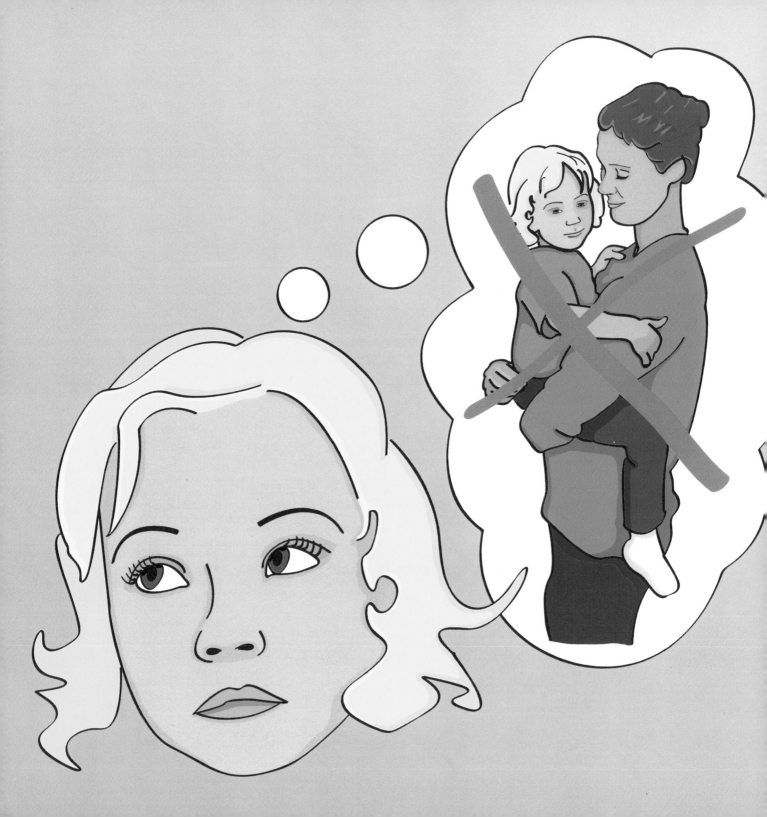

The doctor says mommy is not allowed to pick you up.

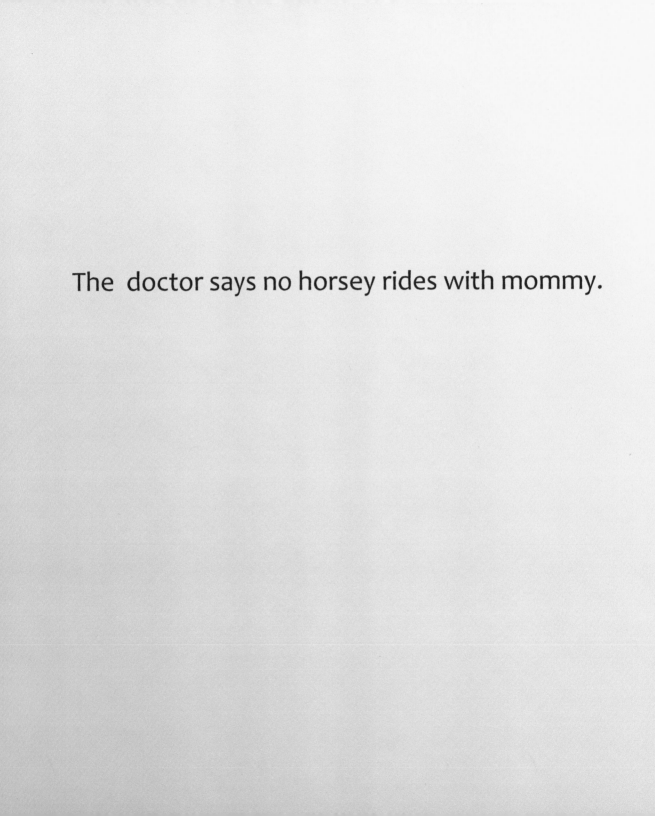

The doctor says no horsey rides with mommy.

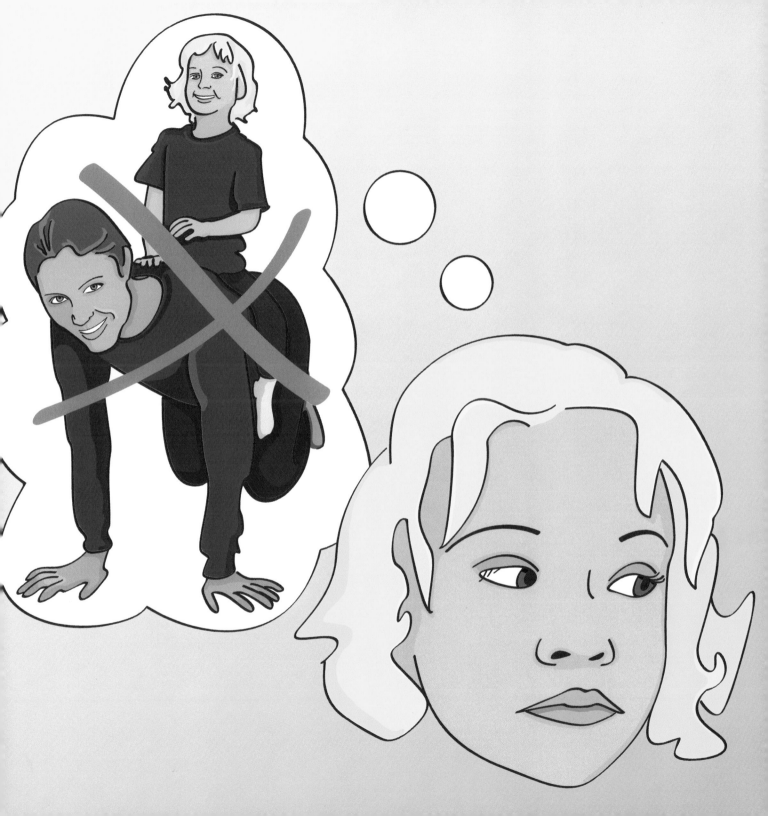

The doctor says
no soccer,
no running,
and no rough play
with mommy.

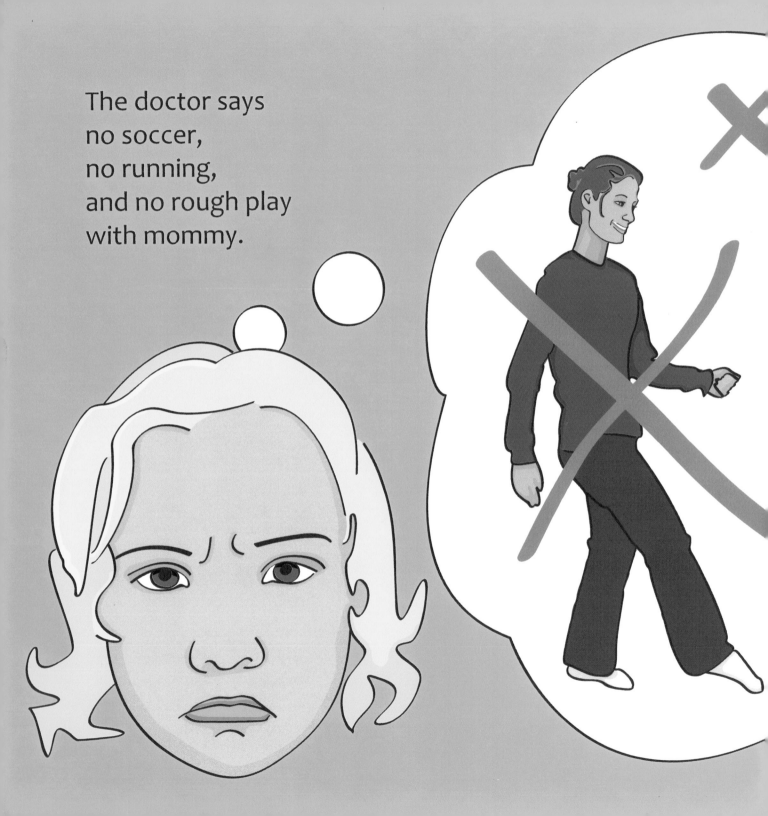

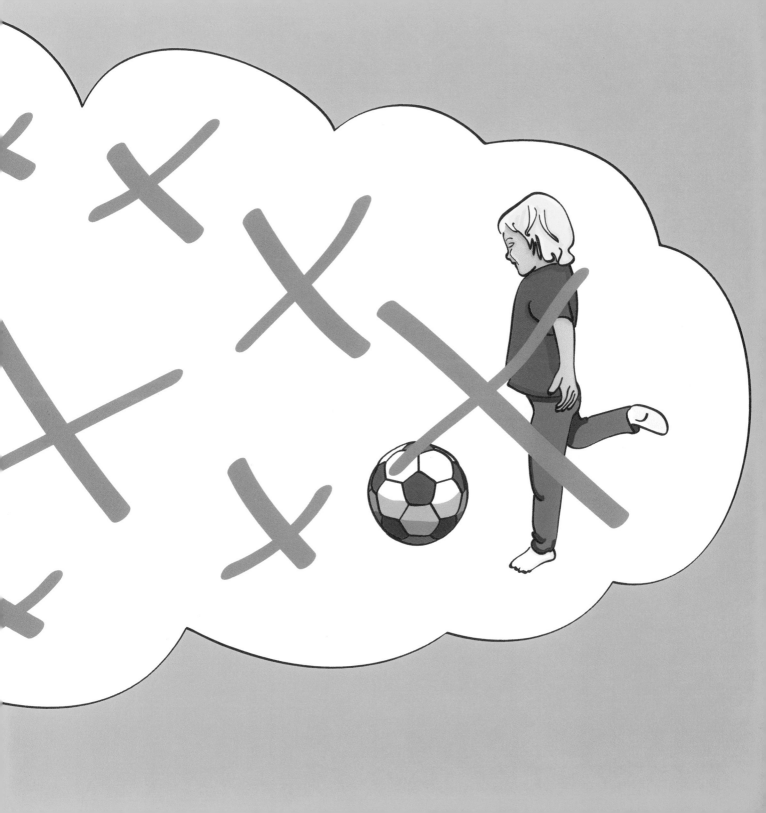

But mommy loves you very much!

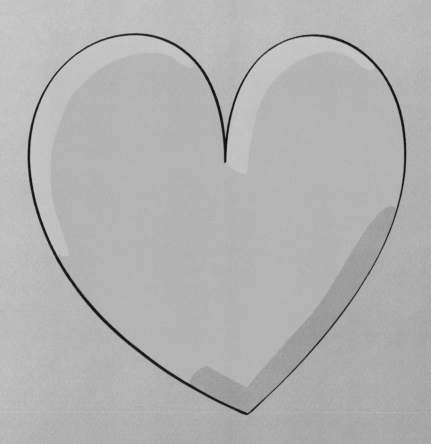

And there are so many things we CAN do with mommy!

We can build a racetrack with mommy.

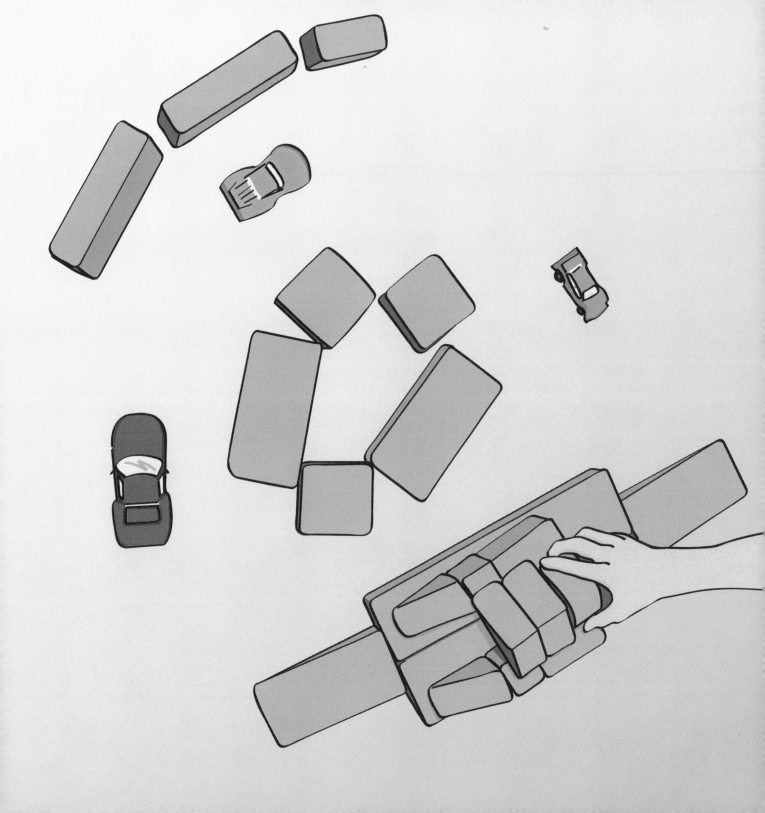

Mommy can play beauty shop.

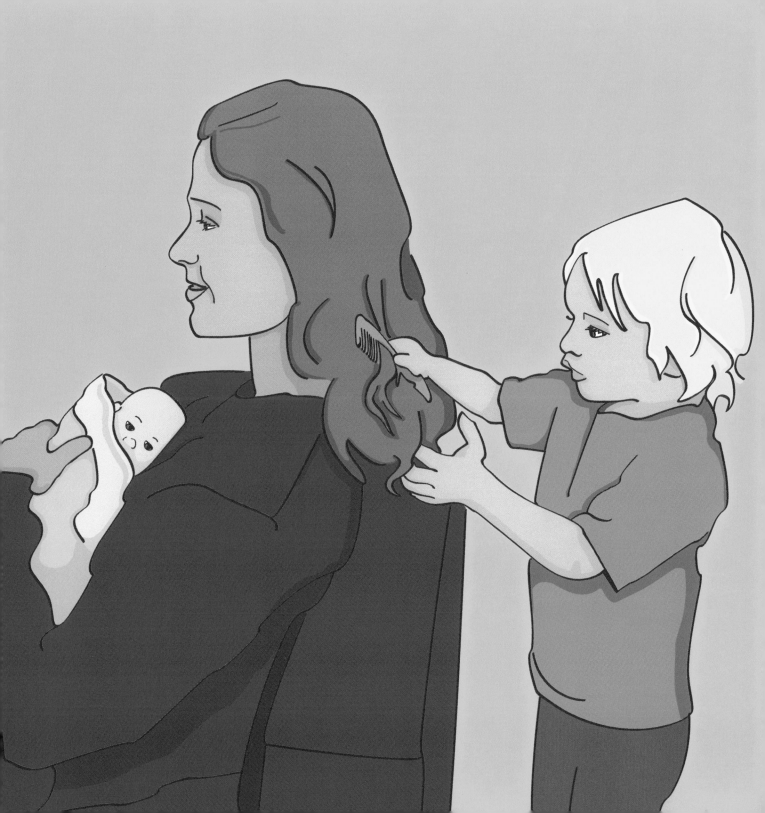

We can put on a puppet show for mommy,

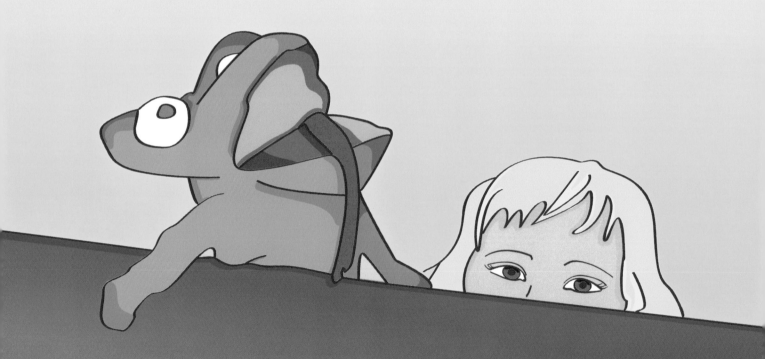

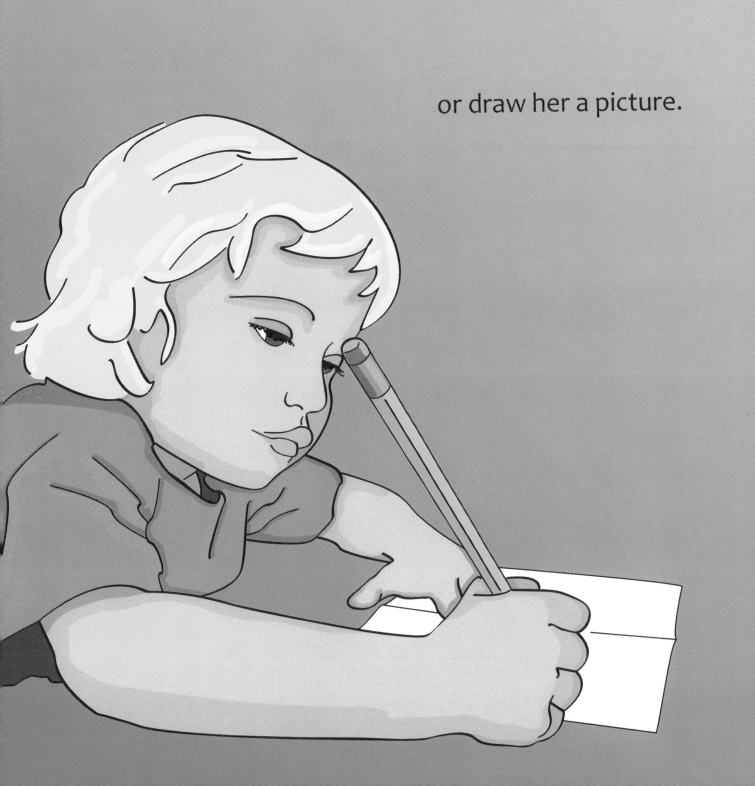

or draw her a picture.

Mommy can build a tower,
play tea party
or create a zoo.

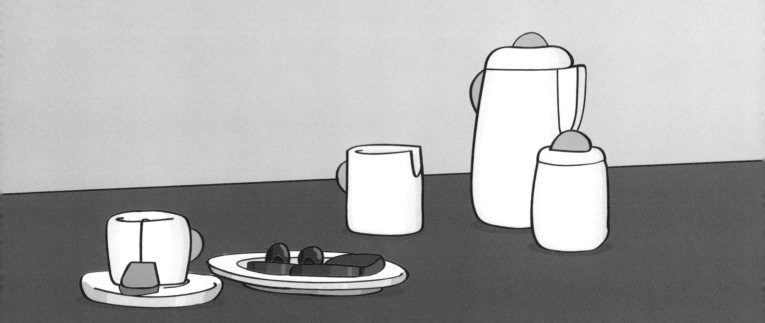

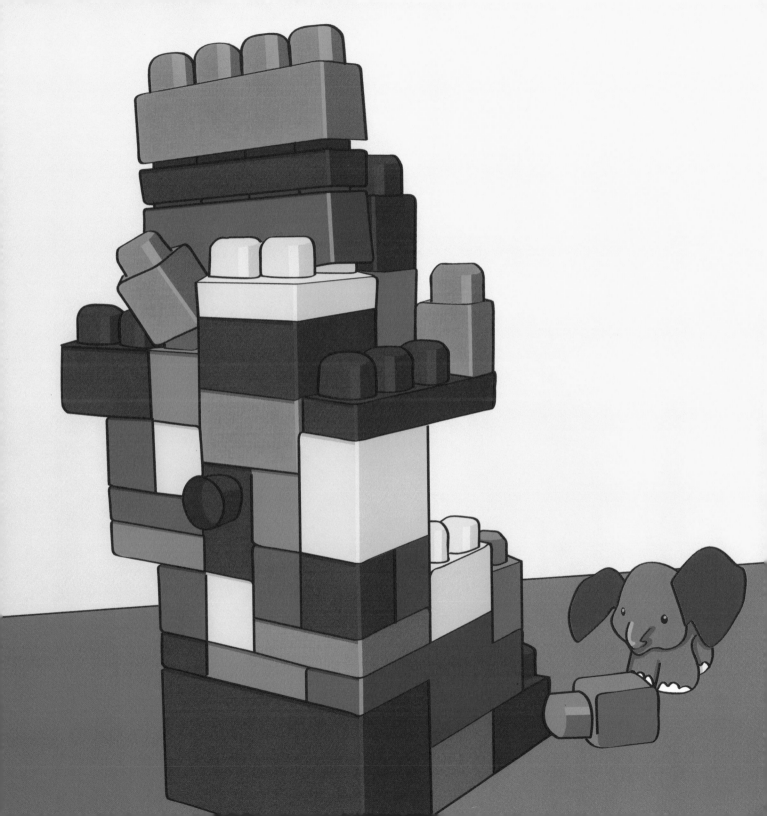

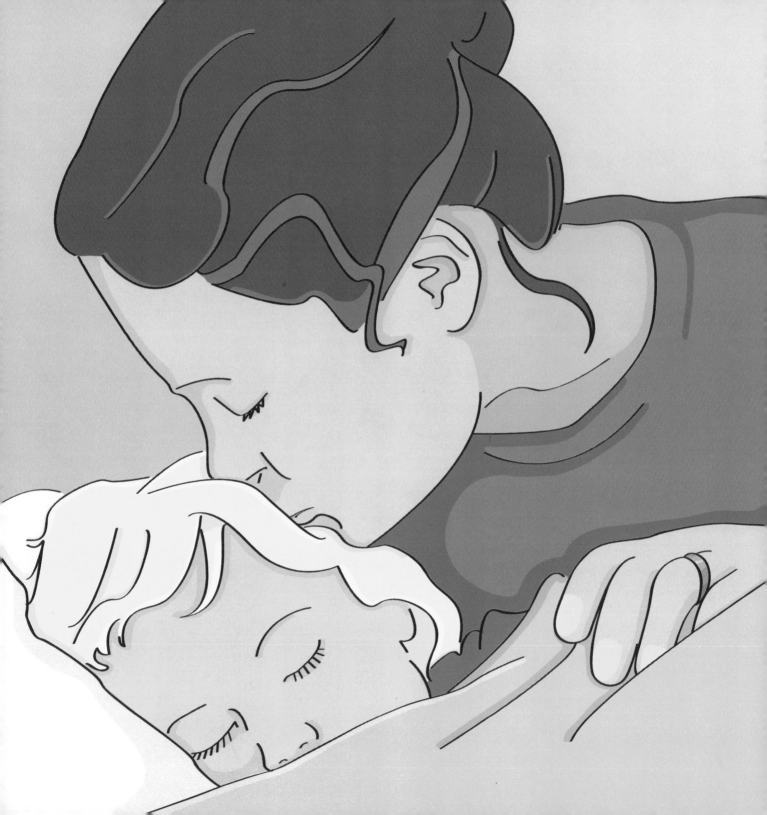

And...

Mommy can tuck you into bed
and kiss you goodnight.

CPSIA information can be obtained
at www.ICGtesting.com
Printed in the USA
271368LV00003B